Positive THINking for weight loss

SHEILA STARR

Good luck
Sheila x

Copyright © 2021 Sheila Starr

All rights reserved.

ISBN: 9798464987005

CONTENTS

	Acknowledgments	i
	Disclaimer	ii
1	Introduction	1
2	Background	Pg 5
3	Step 1 - Decide	Pg 14
4	Step 2 - Exercise	Pg 29
5	Step 3 – Eat Sensibly	Pg 46
6	Step 4 - Planning	Pg 62
7	Step 5 - Celebrate	Pg 70
8	Feel Fabulous	Pg 75
9	Work with Sheila	Pg 80
10	About the Author	Pg 81

ACKNOWLEDGMENTS

Thank you to the inspiring women in my Facebook group, and particular thanks to Pam Reynolds who came up with the name for this book.

DISCLAIMER

I am not a certified Doctor, Dietician or Nutritionist. I do not provide medical or nutrition advice for the purpose of health or disease nor do I claim to be a Doctor, Dietician or Nutritionist. Any recommendation, advice or guidance is not intended to diagnose, treat or cure or prevent any medical ailment or disease. If you do have any medical conditions, please seek professional advice

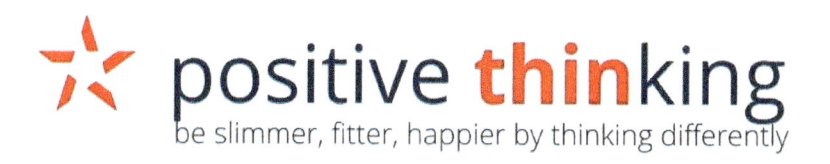

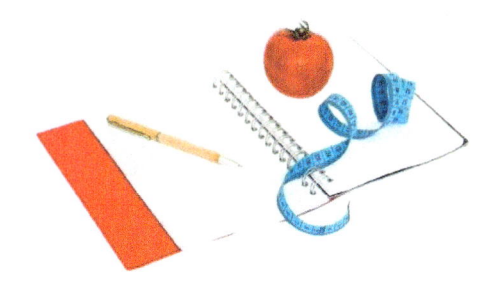

positive thinking
be slimmer, fitter, happier by thinking differently

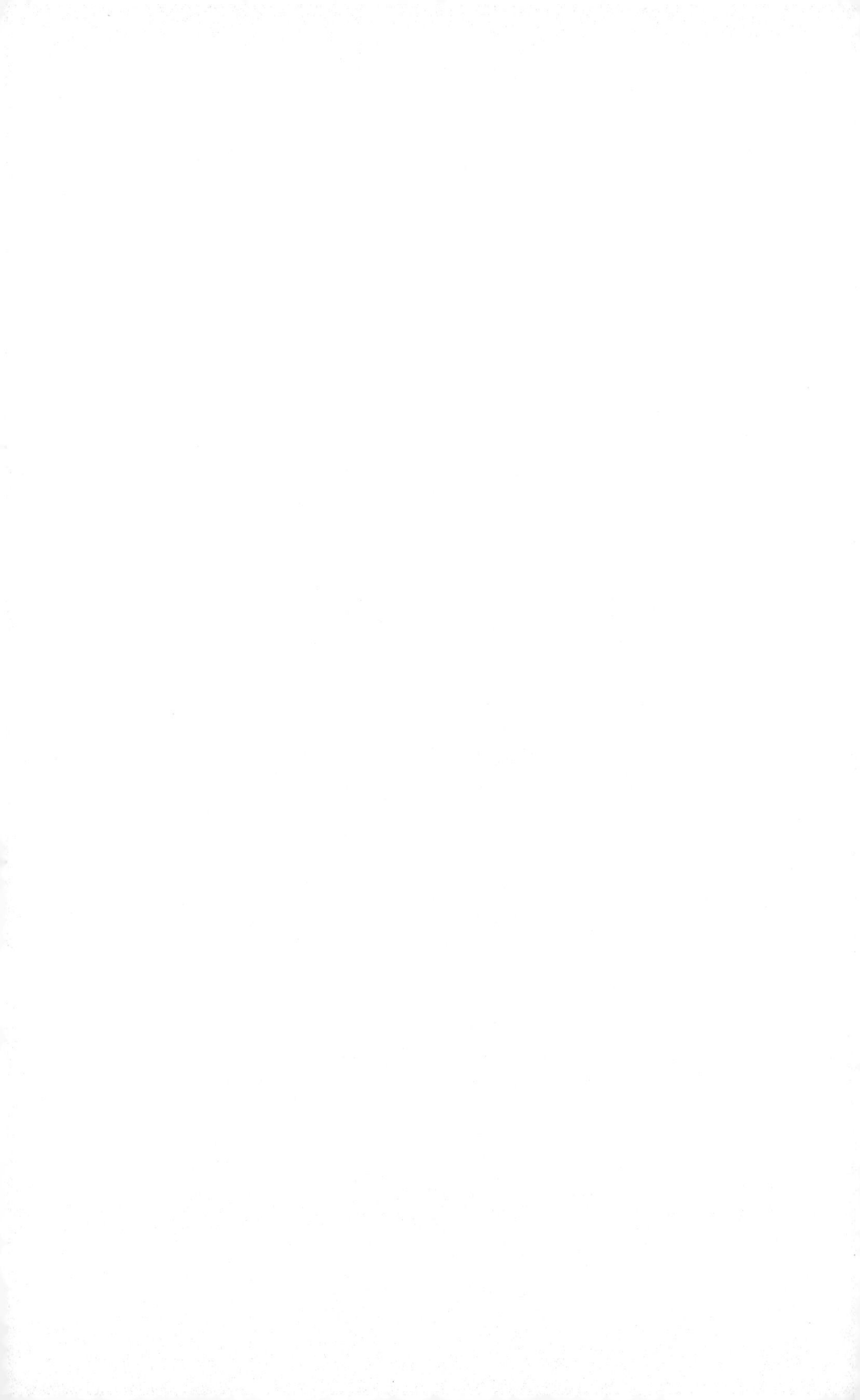

INTRODUCTION

This is a book about how a 50 plus ordinary, busy woman finally conquered her weight and who is now, not only slim and happy with her body, but is also full of energy and feels fabulous.

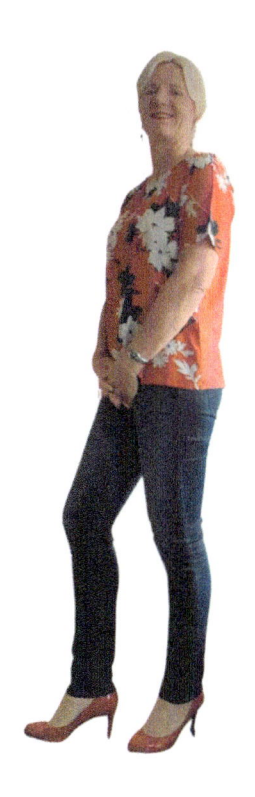

Do you know that **61%** of adults don't like the way they look? I used to be one of them.

Not liking the way we look impacts on our lives so much and yet we really struggle to change ourselves. There are too many temptations in our way, it's so easy to make the wrong choices, and grab a cake instead of an apple.

The shops are against us, they want us to buy their tasty ready meals and sugary snacks, and so they pop them right in our eyeline, it's so hard to resist.

Then others try to persuade us to buy their diet products, foods, slimming clubs, gym memberships. Its big industry, making huge amounts of money and yet we are still all struggling to keep our weight down.

I decided to right this book to help all of you out there, who, like me have spent too many years trying lots of different solutions with little success. Let me be clear, I am just writing about my experience.

I am not a dietician, doctor or expert of any kind. I am a real person, living a real and busy life. I am the person that is bamboozled by jargon and likes things to be very simple.

What this book is and what it isn't.

✓ This book is aimed to inspire you and show you that weight loss does not have to be complicated.

✓ It will share how I made it work for me, an ordinary person with a real and busy life.

✓ It will show you how to make weight loss part of your lifestyle and not be a diet.

✓ It will help you get clear on what you want to achieve and why you want it.

✓ It will show you how to take some simple steps to get started.

× This book will NOT show you how to lose weight quickly, this is a long-term plan.

× It will not talk about nutrients, vitamins and supplements etc.

× It will not address any health issues such as diabetes, allergies etc.

× It will not talk about the science of what you should eat and why.

- ❖ At the end of this book, you will be clear about what you want.

- ❖ You will be committed to achieving it.

- ❖ You will know how to get started.

- ❖ You will understand that it is all about making sensible choices and simply having a positive thinking approach to your lifestyle.

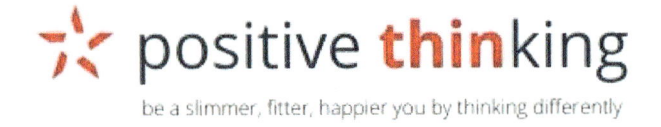

★ positive **thin**king

be a slimmer, fitter, happier you by thinking differently

BACKGROUND

I have been on some kind of diet for over twenty years, and it is exhausting, isn't it?

Actually, BORING is the word that springs to mind. I get so fed up with thinking about food and dieting.

"Is this good for me?"

"How many calories are in that?"

"Should I stop eating carbs?"

"Why is all the tasty food so bad for me?"

"I haven't got time to cook healthy meals"

I have tried all kinds of diet: fasting diets 5:2 / 16:8, detoxes, lean diets, no carb diets, cut out all sugar diets, slimming world, weight watchers, juicing diets.

I have made sure I don't eat after 6pm, always eat breakfast, don't eat processed foods or takeaways, .. well, you know the type of thing.

I have had times when I have declined invitations to go out with friends because I would end up eating something fattening. Then I would get fed up and binge eat on chocolate and hate myself for it.

I bet you feel the same. Do you feel that you have tried everything, and nothing has worked?

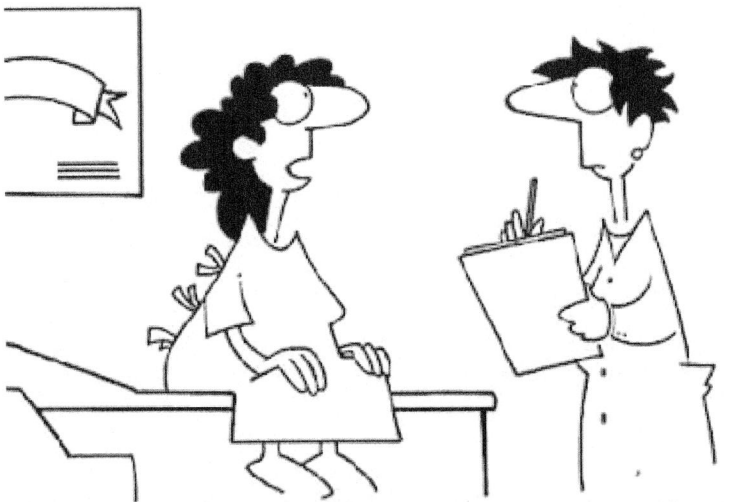

"I have metal fillings in my teeth. My refrigerator magnets keep pulling me into the kitchen. That's why I can't lose weight!"

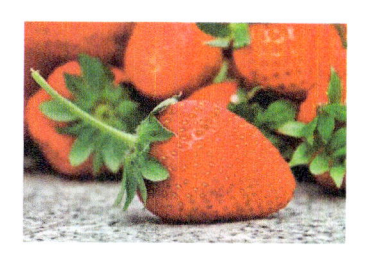

The Food Stuff.

I have never been a great cook; I find it a real faff. I try to cook new recipes but when I open the cookbook or search online, and I see a whole long list of ingredients I get put off.

I don't want to spend my life in the kitchen. Not enjoying cooking means I don't want to spend much time doing it, so I have spent years finding meals that are sensible, healthy enough and quick to make.

If you are like this, then maybe you are turning to ready meals or takeaways too often. Of course, you may have the opposite issue. You may love cooking and baking, maybe you are right at home in the kitchen surrounded by ingredients and recipes.

This is perhaps what is causing you to eat too much of the tasty food you are making and stretching your waistline. Snacking has always been my biggest issue.

Until a few years ago I would have called myself a sugar addict. I loved sweeties and chocolate. I was the person that would buy "3 for a £1" to eat over three days and then eat them all in about ten minutes.

Stopping snacking and reducing my sugar intake has been my single biggest challenge. Do you know what your biggest weakness is? Knowing and acknowledging it is a great first step.

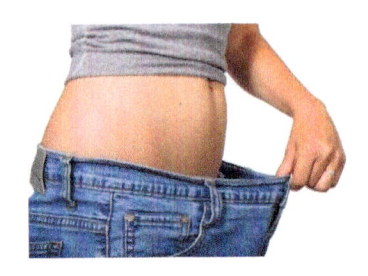

Then There Is The Whole Clothes Situation

I have a wardrobe full of clothes of differing sizes. They start with the "slim me" clothes at one end, move through the "slightly chunky me" clothes and end with the "fat me" clothes at the other end.

For years the "slim me" clothes just sat there gathering dust. Every now and then I'd look at them longingly, then sigh and realise I would never get into them again.

I should give them away, but I didn't, because we live in hope, don't we? We think just maybe, one day, I'll get into them again.

Perhaps we are delusional but maintaining hope is a good thing, don't give up that dream of wearing those skinny jeans again.

I would open my wardrobe and hate everything in it, because the nice clothes didn't fit, and the clothes that fit didn't make me feel nice. So, I'd pull out the same old outfit that I always did and feel fat, frumpy and frustrated.

I am so glad that I hung on to my "slim me" clothes because I am now wearing them again.

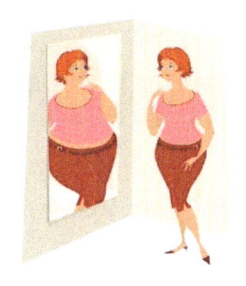

The Misery of The Mirror

For a while I lived in a rented flat that didn't have a full-length mirror and it was quite liberating.

Of course, it didn't change the fact that I was fatter than I wanted to be, but it did take away the misery of seeing my body in its full glory.

Do you hate seeing your body in the mirror, but can't help but look? It's like a gory scene from a car crash, you want to look but you don't want to, so you turn your head partly away and glance at it sideways.

Every morning for many years I would see myself in the mirror and hate my body. I would hate my bingo wings, my wobbly thighs, my chubby cheeks.

It didn't lead to a very positive start to the day. I had low self-esteem and was lacking in confidence, all because of how I looked.

Eventually the mirror became my friend and my motivation to make a lasting change.

A Bit About Me

In my thirties I started to put on weight gradually, so it wasn't very noticeable to other people.

I wasn't doing any exercise anymore, not out dancing in clubs, not so many activity-based hobbies. It was all about socialising, eating, drinking, cinema etc.

I have never been obese. I am quite tall and carry my weight well. When I put on weight, it goes on all over and so doesn't appear out of proportion. I also dress to hide the flab; I wear heels that gives me more height.

Other people would not call me fat; whenever I would refuse a cake, they would say "you don't need to lose weight, you look fine". That was not helpful, as I would believe them.

I am 5 foot 7 inches, and at my heaviest I was 13 stone. I was buying size 16 clothes. I wanted to be under 11 stone, as long as it started with a 10, I didn't mind if it was 10'13 and to get back into a size 12.

It seemed impossible though. I would tell myself that I am not twenty, it's inevitable that I'll be heavier, isn't it? Over the last ten years I have consistently weighed between 12 and 13 stone.

I have done regular exercise which has kept me from gaining even more weight. Until the 2020 pandemic, I went to the gym every weekday for ten years and either swam or used the cardio equipment. I have two friends who I met there, which kept me turning up, but the focus was lacking and occasionally we even just had a shower and a coffee.

So, What Changed?

Well, a couple of things:

One day in November 2019 when I stood in front of the mirror, something snapped, and I decided enough was enough and I had to make a change.

Then the voice in my head said "Ah, it's almost Christmas, let's wait until the new year" but as I said it, I realised that this wasn't acceptable. I had a word with myself, it was still 5 weeks until Christmas and I could lose half a stone by then. So, that's what I did.

The other thing that changed was my environment. I was made redundant in January 2020 and then when the pandemic hit, it created an opportunity for me to try something different.

I know a lot of people spent lockdown baking and drinking and so gained a few lockdown pounds. But I started walking every day. Over the course of 8 months, I gradually found things that really worked for me, that I could make a habit and that became part of my lifestyle.

No more feeling like I was missing out or doing things I didn't really want to do. I loved what I was doing, and I didn't just lose weight, I felt amazing. I started to love myself again, I felt more confident, more productive. I had more energy, I slept better, and I felt happy.

I LOST 2 AND A HALF STONE IN 8 MONTHS AND HAVE MAINTAINED THAT WEIGHT LOSS.

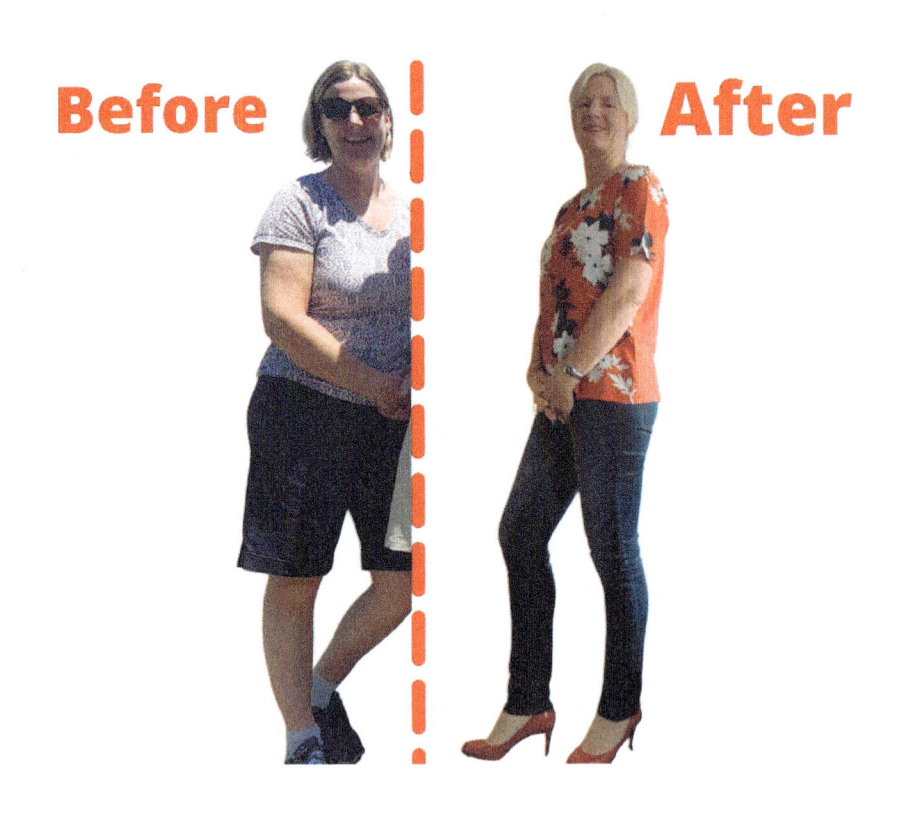

In this book I will share with you the five steps that not only helped me lose weight but improved both my physical and mental wellbeing.

THE TRUTH ABOUT WEIGHT LOSS IS THAT ITS ALL IN THE MIND

* It doesn't matter which diet you try, if your mind is not in the right place you will fail.

* It doesn't matter which diet you try, if your mind is in the right place you will succeed.

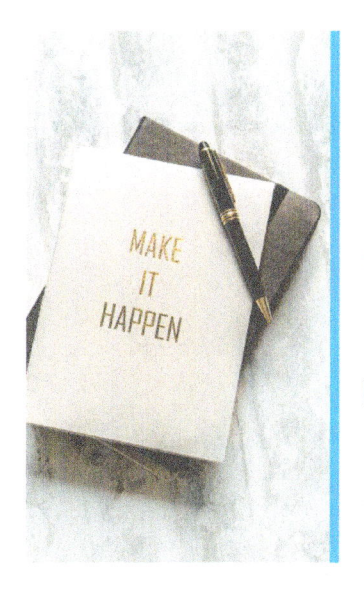

"If you really want to do something, you'll find a way.

If you don't, you'll find an excuse."

Jim Rohn

Which is why the first step in this process is to **DECIDE**

STEP 1 - DECIDE

Choose to lose

It is all about your mindset, how you learn to think differently. Whatever you do, don't skip this step as without changing your mindset you won't change anything else. Nothing will work for you if your mind is not set in the right way. I am not pretending this will be easy, but this is the bit to spend your time and focus on

Whether you think you CAN
or
you think you CAN'T
You are right

Henry Ford

Remember, the only person stopping you lose weight is

YOU

As I see it, you have three options:

1) You don't change anything, and you remain unhappy with yourself.

2) You choose to love yourself just the way you are.

3) You DECIDE to make a positive change and become the person you are proud to be.

Let's just have a look at those three options:

1) If you **don't change** anything:

You will always be disappointed with yourself; you will lack energy and confidence. You will continue to compare yourself to others wishing you could be slim like they are. You will hate all your clothes; you will avoid looking in the mirror and you will judge yourself poorly.

You might miss out on things because you don't feel good enough to step up and apply for that promotion, date that handsome man, meet new friends.

This is about so much more than just losing weight. This is about you learning to love yourself again, be kind to yourself and be proud of yourself. This is about understanding that you are good enough and that you deserve to be healthy and happy.

2) Choosing to *love yourself* just the way you are:

This is powerful and at some stage in this process that is exactly what you will be doing. This a huge mindset shift and I am guessing that because you are reading this book, you haven't found a way to love yourself yet.

We often compare ourselves to others and that makes us constantly dissatisfied with ourselves. Don't worry about anyone else, just set your own standards and aim for those. Be who you want to be and recognise when you have got there.

3) DECIDING to make a *positive change*:

This is going to improve your life significantly, and once you really have decided and committed to it, you will find a way. This book will help you find a way that works for you and makes it a lifestyle change rather than a diet.

But DECIDING isn't easy.

Maybe you have had an epiphany or a breakthrough moment where you have realised that NOW is the time, and you are determined to make a change. Perhaps you are just constantly looking for the thing that's going to work for you.

Whatever your reasons DECIDING is the first step. But I bet you have decided before, got committed and somehow it didn't work out, or maybe you did lose weight but now its gradually going back on again.

Do you find excuses why it hasn't worked before?

You believe you haven't got any willpower, or that you are naturally heavy boned.

You are definitely telling yourself that you haven't got TIME:

*Not enough time to cook healthy meals from scratch

OR

*Not enough time to fit in any exercise.

Maybe you think you haven't got enough MONEY:

*Not enough money to cook healthy meal

OR

*Not enough money to join the gym, go to a class, buy any kit

None of this is true, it is just what you are telling yourself.

We need to work on removing those limiting beliefs and create some new empowering beliefs.

QUESTION:

How much do you like yourself?

I don't just mean how you look but how much do you like yourself as a person?

Are you kind to yourself or are you always telling yourself how rubbish you are? Do you tell yourself how awesome you are, or how you could do better?

Do you want to be more confident, more ambitious, more adventurous? Do you want to feel happy and fulfilled?

It helps if you like yourself. Write a list of all the things you do like about yourself.

Maybe you are generous, caring, lively, cheerful, positive. Perhaps you are good at problem solving, seeing the good in others, listening.

Only think about the things you like about yourself. Ask you friends and family what they like about you. Other people always see us differently, they will see more of the good in you that you do in yourself. Every day, focus on what you like about yourself rather than what you don't like.

You need be kind to yourself and know you deserve to look and feel better, then change will come.

"Why would you improve the life

of someone you don't like?"

Sheila Starr

Your notes: write here what you like about yourself

If you crack the mindset piece, then the rest becomes easy. Spend some time on this, it will be worth it.

Let me walk you through a process to get you fully committed to losing weight and loving yourself.

I want you to look in the mirror and SMILE at the awesome person looking back at you.

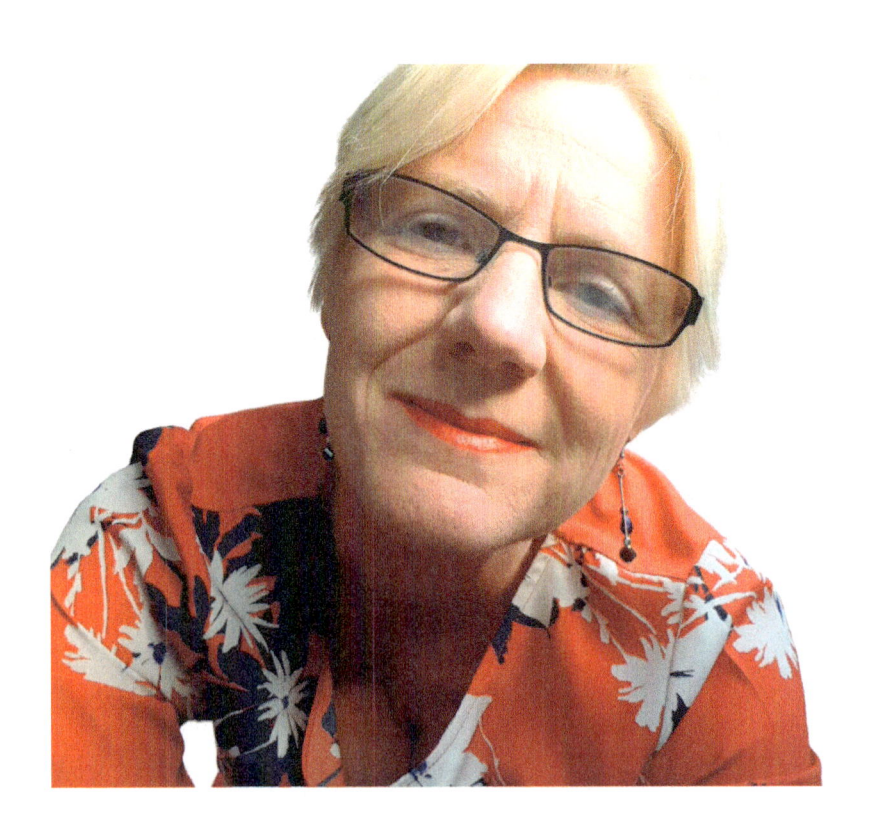

WHAT?

Firstly, understand WHAT it is you want to achieve, be specific.

It's not good enough to say, "I want to lose weight". You need some clarity about what you want to achieve. You need a good old target to aim for, if you don't have a target, you can't see what progress you are making.

So, what is your target? Here are some examples:

*I want to lose 2 stone before my holiday next summer

*I want to lose 5 stone in 2 years

*I want to get into my posh dress in time for my friend's wedding

*I want to lose 1 stone before my daughters' sports day

You get the idea, so take a moment and think about what your target is.

You do need to be realistic about what you can achieve, so be careful here with your timescales.

You won't lose a stone in a week, and it would be unhealthy to do so. Everything takes longer than you think it will, so keep the pressure off and give yourself time. You are in this for the long haul, for sustainable results.

Your "**what**": write your goal here

WHY?

OK, so you know WHAT you want to achieve, that's a great start but WHY do you want to achieve it?

Your WHY is the reason you will achieve it.

This is the part where you really COMMIT to your goal and that's what makes the difference between losing weight and not losing weight.

This is where you delve deeply into yourself and find an emotional reason WHY you want to lose weight. This is NOT about why you SHOULD lose weight. This not about WISHING you could lose weight and it is definitely NOT about what other people thing you should do. This is about why YOU want to lose weight.

You need to have a really strong WHY, a really powerful reason why you want to lose weight. If you don't then it's very unlikely that you will lose weight, you just don't want it enough. So, find an emotional connection with your weight, dig deep and understand how being overweight is impacting on your life.

Think about the negative impact being overweight is having on your life.

What pain is it causing? What is it stopping you from doing?

*Do you hate seeing yourself in the mirror?

*Have you outgrown all your clothes?

*Are you embarrassed when you meet the parents of your children's friends?

*Is it stopping you going out and socialising?

*Are you out of breath when you climb up the stairs?

*Can you not bend down to pick up your dog's ball?

*Are you scared that being overweight will cause poor health and an early death.

Your "pain": write your notes here.

What would your life be like if you lost weight?

*Would you smile when you saw yourself in the mirror?

*Would you be able to wear all your favourite clothes again?

*Would you apply for that new job you saw advertised?

*Would you go on a beach holiday and wear your bikini?

*Would you enjoy running around the garden with your children?

When you think about the impact being overweight is having on your life and the impact it would have if you lost the weight, feel it. Really get emotionally attached to the impact it's having on your life.

If you are not feeling emotional about it, if you can't find a WHY that you really connect with, then you don't want it enough. This is why nothing has worked before, and why it won't work this time. Dig deeper, try again, what is it you really want and why do you want it.

If you have found your WHY, you will now start to be feel determined to reach your goal. Once you know your WHY and you get fully committed to achieving it, you will do it. You will find a way.

My Why was twofold. I hated seeing my reflection every day, looking at my pale flabby body when I got dressed was depressing. Plus, I was so fed up with thinking about it all the time. I spent so much time and energy hating myself, planning my food, fitting in exercise, it was tiresome.

Then there is the disappointment, when you give up on the diet and exercise and scoff some sugary, tasty, fattening food. I had let myself down again!

That day in November was my turning point. It was the day that my WHY became stronger than my love of eating.

It was D Day – **Determination**.

I now knew **what** I wanted to achieve – to get back into my size 12 skinny jeans.

I knew **why** – to be happy and proud when I looked in the mirror

I just needed to find a way to get started. For me snacking was my biggest problem, so I started by cutting out sugary snacks. That's what I needed to kickstart my weight loss.

What is your "why"?

Your "why" write your why here

VISUALISATION

Visualisation can be really powerful if you practice and really believe in it. It is a method that sees you delve deep with your mind and emotions and look at what it is you want to achieve.

In my online course I share a couple of short visualisations that you can use to help. Here I will explain how it works and you can design your own.

Find yourself a quiet space where you are comfortable, and you won't be interrupted. Allow just 5 minutes and close your eyes (once you have read this, obviously).

Now, imagine yourself as you would like to look. Be specific, what dress size are you wearing, how does your face look, have your bingo wings reduced, how big is your bum? What clothes are you wearing? What style is your hair? Are you at a party having fun with friends and getting yourself in every photo shot?

What does it feel like to be this version of you? Properly feel it, are you smiling more, do you have more energy, is life more fun?

Hang on to this feeling and practice this visualisation every day. The more you can really imagine yourself looking like that, the more you will be committed to achieving it.

Now, this may seem odd but before we move on to more practical tips, I really need you to be determined to change your body, so……

Undress and stand in front of a full-length mirror.

Take a look at yourself, notice all the wobbly bits, the fat, the things you really hate about your body. I want you to feel how much you hate your body, how embarrassed you are, how emotional you feel when you see yourself.

Take a selfie (maybe with underwear on), print it off and write on it, how you feel being that person, how much you hate being that person. Write it so that when you look at it again, you feel the emotion that you feel right now.

Keep this photo somewhere you see it, this will come in very useful when you are struggling to stay committed to losing weight.

Whenever you have a day where you want to give in and eat cake – look at this photo and think "I don't want to be that person anymore"

Then revisit the visualisation of the new you and renew your determination to make the change.

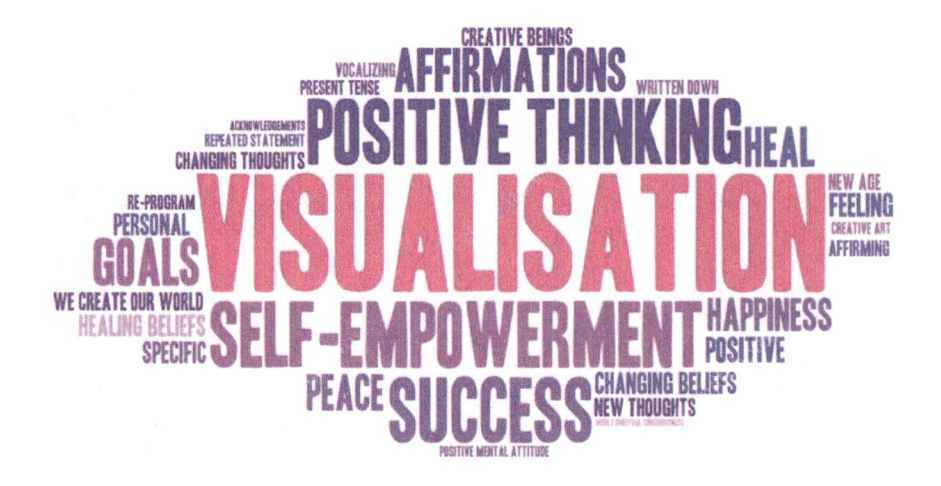

STEP 2 - EXERCISE

Move More

Lots of people get hung up on the exercise part of losing weight but it is essential. The trick is to find some form of exercise that you enjoy, that doesn't feel like a chore, and that fits into your life easily.

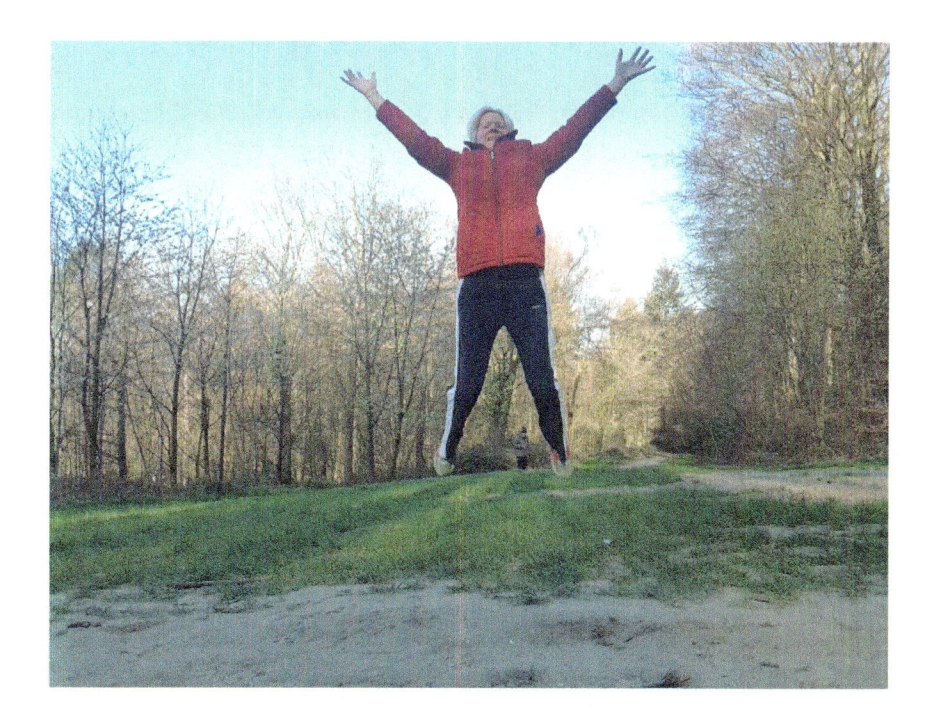

We have very sedentary lives these days, there is a lot of sitting down involved. The less you move, the less you want to move and so the less we do move.

My first tip is to just: **MOVE MORE**

Just notice how much you are sitting down and get up and move about.

Not only will moving more burn a few calories but it will also improve your mood, your energy and your performance.

If you are sitting at a desk all day, firstly check your posture, don't slump, sitting up straight will help you feel less stressed. It will also keep you more alert and therefore more focussed and productive.

Make sure you regularly get up and walk around. Walk to the kitchen, the bathroom, or anywhere, just walk somewhere. Walk with purpose and energy, stand tall and stride it out.

Set an alarm, if you need to, to ensure that you remember to get up and move. When you are sitting watching tv, have a good fidget. Then get up in between each programme and stretch your legs, give your body a shake down, a wiggle.

If you make a cup of tea do a few laps of the kitchen while the kettle boils.

Whenever you have a few minutes, instead of scrolling through social media pop on a tune and have a dance. I love a good bop around my kitchen, I really let go and enjoy myself. Occasionally, mid bop, I realise my husband is standing in the doorway watching me with a grin on his face.

The point is to find ways to add movement to your day. The more you move the fitter you will be both physically and mentally. The more you move the better you will feel and the more energy you will have.

What could you do to move more? Write your notes here.........

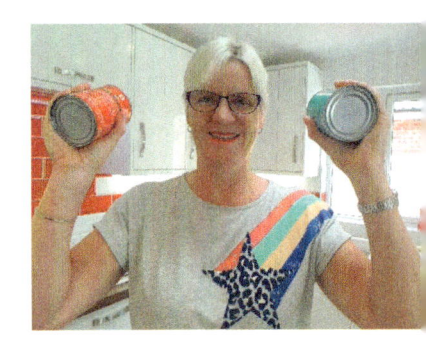

TIME HACK

For those of you that believe you don't have enough time to fit in exercise – this is for you.

Do exercises while cooking your dinner. You could burn off 100 calories while you are cooking.

*Take two tins of beans (or any other tins) and do some arm curls

*March on the spot lifting your knees as high as you can, start slow, and get faster.

*Jog on the spot if you are able .

*Do some squats, balance using the work surface .

*Put on lively music and have a dance.

Other ways to fit exercise in:

*Park further away from the shops/office.

*When you are cleaning the house, put more physical effort into it, dance the hoover round.

*Do squats or march when you are cleaning your teeth

EXERCISE

Master It

OK, so let's talk about exercise. If you want to lose weight, you really do need to do some kind of exercise. You need to find something that you enjoy so much that you want to do it and it becomes part of your lifestyle.

Finding something you want to master turns it from being something you have to do to something you want to do. The feeling of satisfaction when you improve at a skill is incredible.

For me, it used to be swimming. I used to get up early and head to the leisure centre before work. Over ten years I became a pretty good swimmer. I started off in the slow lane, doing breaststroke with my head above the water, and progressed to the fast crawl lane, swimming at least a mile every day. I was able to swim longer distances and my times got quicker, and I had a sense of pride.

Swimming is a great exercise, its kind to your joints and works a lot of your muscles, maybe it's something you want to try.

I tried running one year, someone told me I'd love running so I gave it a go. I didn't! Love it, that is. In fact, I hated it, the only thing I liked about it was stopping.

I did run a 5k and a 10k that year, so I proved I could run, but why would I if I hated it.

I've been the person that goes to the gym every day, treadmills, exercise bikes, cross trainers but even though I was committed to going every day, the effort wasn't always put in.

I never really liked the gym, I went because I wanted to keep my weight down, or rather, that I didn't want to put on any more weight. So, even though I was either swimming or going to the gym every weekday, my weight wasn't where I wanted it to be. Partly due to the fact that you can't out train a bad diet and I had a bad diet, and also because just showing up at the gym, unfortunately, doesn't burn calories without the effort.

When the Covid 19 pandemic hit, the leisure centre closed, and I had to find a different way to exercise. For me, it was walking. That's it, just walking. It doesn't cost anything, I don't need any gym membership or kit, just a pair of trainers. Oh, I do also wear a sports bra, but you may not need to.

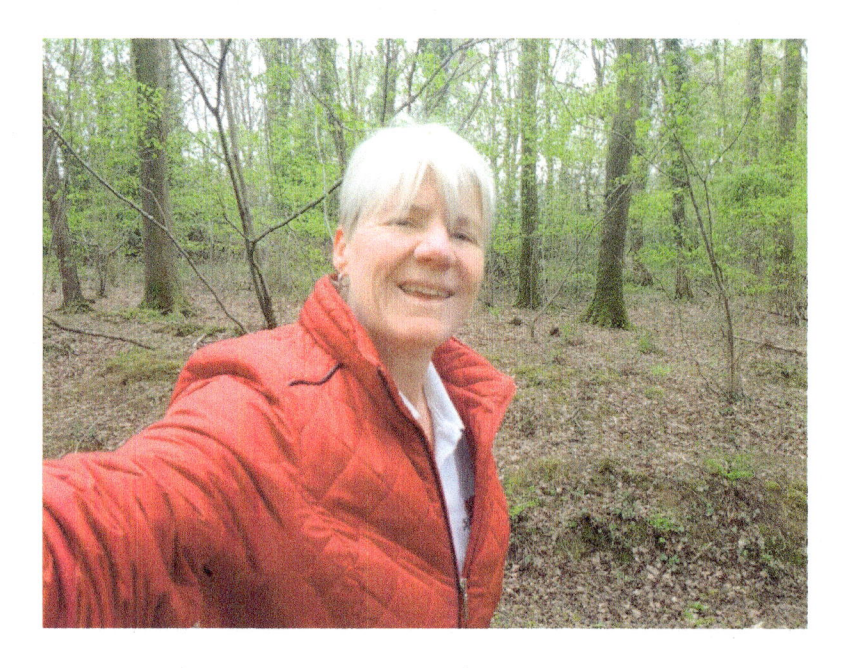

WALK YOURSELF SLIM

I started walking in the woods at the start of the Covid pandemic in March 2020. The leisure centre closed, I was working from home, and I needed to not only get some exercise, but I craved a change of scenery. So, I found an entrance to the local woods and started walking there every day.

You may be thinking, it's OK for you, you work for yourself, you don't have any children to deal with, I don't have time to fit in a walk, or a swim etc

Not having time is a great excuse, but you do have time. You make time for the things you want to do. When I was working in corporate life, I got up at 5.30 to go for a swim. I still get up early to fit in my walk. You might need to do your exercise at lunch time or maybe once the kids have gone to bed.

I would also argue that if you haven't got time, then maybe other self-care aspects are missing from your life and actually, in order to have a healthy life, you MUST find time to look after yourself. Prioritise your wellbeing – this comes back to how much you like yourself enough to care for you.

Although I don't have children, I do have a disabled husband to care for. This is why walking in the morning works for me, as he is asleep in bed and doesn't miss me or need me in the early hours of the morning.

Walking helped me become healthier both physically and mentally.

It gave me space to be with my own thoughts and ideas but also to remove myself from my life for a short while and just mindfully enjoy the wonder of nature.

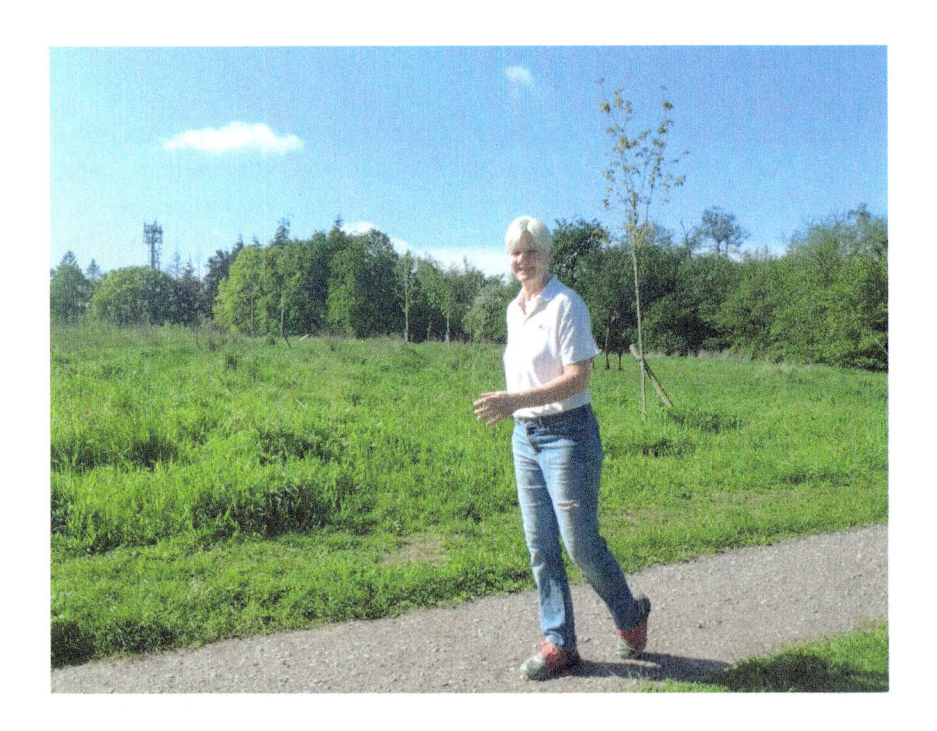

Benefits of walking

* Walking one mile burns approximately 100 calories.

* It tones your legs, particularly if you find some inclines or hills.

* It will tone your arms if you swing them purposefully while walking, any help with the bingo wings gratefully received!

* It eases joint pain and helps prevent arthritis.

* It strengthens your heart and reduces heart disease by 20%.

* It boosts your energy by increasing the level of hormones that elevate energy levels. Apparently its better than a cup of coffee at giving you're an energy boost.

* It boosts your immune system, reducing the chances of catching a cold or flu.

*It improves your mood, helps reduce anxiety and stress and boosts your self-esteem.

* It creates a change of environment, which in 2020 was vital due to being locked down in our own homes.

* It helps with problem solving and creative thinking by clearing your head and encouraging a free flow of ideas.

Wow, look at all of those benefits, just from going out for a walk.

How to walk with weight loss in mind

* Walk with purpose, this walk isn't a nice stroll in the park, it's to help you lose weight.

* Walk at a good pace, get your heart pumping.

* Walk upright, shoulders back but relaxed.

* Swing your arms in a controlled way to help tone your arms as well, this will also burn a few more calories.

* Aim for a 20-minute mile to start with, and then as you get fitter gradually increase your speed. You are aiming for a 17-minute mile, this is fast enough to make you fitter but not so fast that you miss the enjoyment of the walk.

*Aim for a minimum of 2 miles, that's 40 minutes each day. If you have time then walk further, the more you walk the more weight your will lose. Each mile is approximately 2000 steps.

If you don't have much time for your walk, you could incorporate some HIIT sections to your walk. This is when you spend two minutes walking as fast as you physically can, then two minutes at a medium pace, then back to the fast pace again. Do this for 10 minutes a couple of times on your walk.

Try and walk every day, even if you only do one mile.

How to enjoy your walk

* Find somewhere nice to walk, a local park, the woods, the seafront. If you don't have these nearby, then find interesting residential roads to walk down, ones with less traffic.

* Notice your surroundings. Properly see what is around you whether it's the squirrels, birds, trees, flowers, dogs running, children playing or the type of cars on driveways.

* Smile at the wind in your hair, the sun on your face, the raindrops on your head.

* Engage with other people you see, just smile and say hello, maybe comment on their dog or the weather.

* Explore new routes, find paths you have never been down before, seek out new places to discover.

* If you are an earbud sort of person, you can use your walk to learn something, a self-help podcast or learn a language, or just listen to some music.

* You could find a friend to walk with. Having a buddy can help you commit to going out but choose someone who wants to help you get fit, not someone who is going to slow you down, or persuade you to go for coffee and cake instead.

How to improve your mental health when walking

* Use the space to think through any issues you have with a positive mindset, this is the time to find constructive solutions to challenges (if you find yourself dwelling on something negative -stop yourself and turn it into a positive approach).

* Find a moment of calm, somewhere you can stop and just "be" for a moment, banish all thoughts and just breathe in the wonder of life.

* Use affirmations to boost your self-esteem and train your brain that you are capable of amazing things (there are plenty of examples online)

* Ensure that your body is relaxed and not tight, lower your shoulders, lift your head, smile.

* Get out of your own head for a while, stop any thoughts and just focus on your walk.

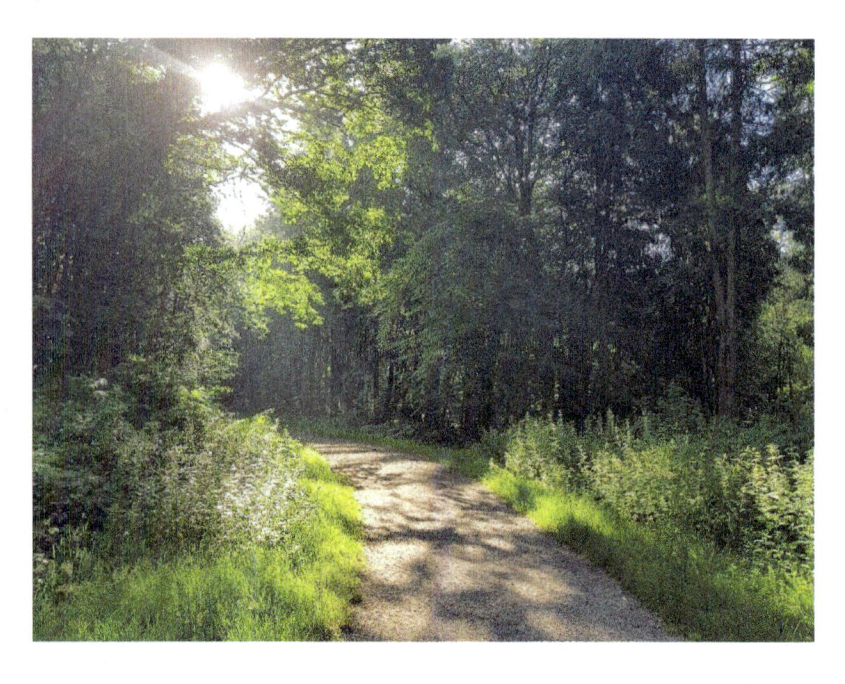

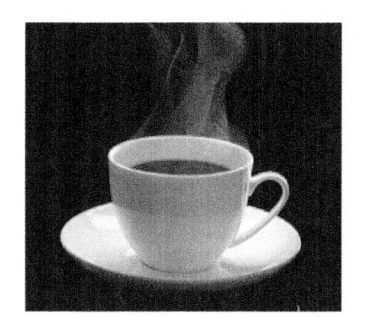

Rewards

It's always good to reward yourself for taking action. For me the enjoyment of being out in nature is reward enough, I look forward to my walks. But your reward could be:

* A nice warm shower when you get back.

* A hot mug of steaming coffee.

* The satisfying ache of your muscles.

* Watching an episode of A Place in the Sun, or whatever tv show you use for escapism.

* A hug from your children.

Perhaps you want to track your exercise and your reward is seeing the consistency of your action, or that your walk was longer or faster than last time.

I use MapMy Walk app, to track my walks, I love seeing the map of my walk after its loaded, the elevations, the pace of each mile. It motivates me to stick to my goal of 5 miles every day, which is 10,000 steps.

I have a story about how I came to walk 5 miles every day. When I started walking in lockdown I was doing 5 Kilometres each day. I figured that's what people ran so it felt like a good aim. I had time and I could easily walk that distance in the woods without retracing my steps or doing loops.

There were days where I would walk more, 6 or 7k, and that made me feel like an overachiever. Then, I was talking to a friend about how I had adapted my exercise after the leisure centre closing and he asked me, how many steps that was. I had no idea; I hadn't looked at steps.

Well, 5k is 7500 steps and that made me rethink my goals. It has always been the recommendation to walk 10,000 steps each day and I wasn't. During lockdown, I was hardly doing any steps as I wasn't going anywhere, and our house isn't big enough for many steps. We haven't even got any stairs as we live in a bungalow, so I worked out how far I'd need to walk to do 10,000 steps and it was 8k.

My husband was always asking me how many miles I had walked but my app was in kilometres. So, I changed the setting in the app to miles and set out to do 10,000 steps, which is 5 miles.

Now I walk 5 miles every day, unless it's absolutely pouring with rain and then I don't!

The message I want you to hear is that you don't need to go to the gym or a class in order to do exercise. You don't need to do something you don't like doing to get moving more. Find something that works for you but **do something.**

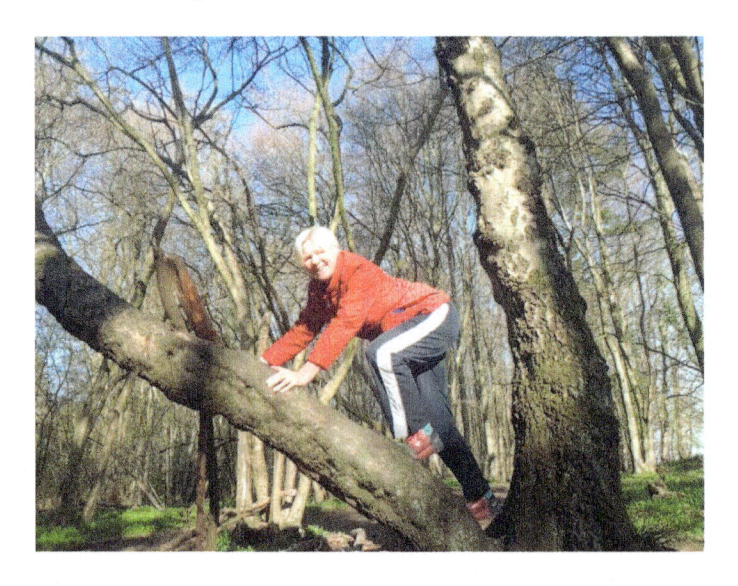

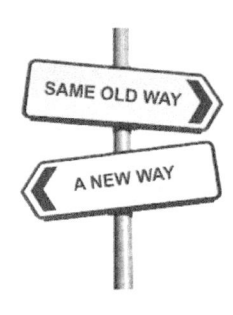

Make it a habit

Once you have identified what sort of movement or exercise works for you, you need to make it a habit. This is much easier if you have found something that you enjoy doing and want to improve at.

My personal opinion and experience is that habits are made easily if you do it every day, at least to start with. If I miss a day, or say I am going to do it every other day, I have always failed.

In order for my brain to move into automatic mode, it needs to be trained to do exercise every day. Its like cleaning my teeth. I do it every day, I don't even think about it, I just do it. I never think "I'm too busy", " I cant be bothered", my brain just knows it has to do it.

So, if you decide you really want to lose weight, then I'd highly recommend that you do some kind of exercise every day, and at the same time.

Habits are formed by doing the same thing, at the same time consistently.

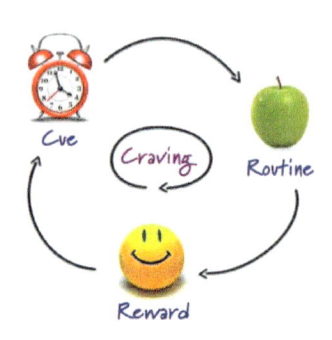

Creating a habit has a formula

Cue – Routine – Reward

You need a cue or a trigger to get you started, so for me, it's getting up in the morning. As soon as I wake up, I get dressed and go for my walk (after going to the toilet and cleaning my teeth, of course)

For you, it might be, when your alarm goes off, when you finish work for the day, when the kids have gone to bed. Find a trigger that your brain will identify with.

The routine is just doing it consistently. Do it every day. There are various views on how many times it takes to make it a habit, 21 days, 28 days, 3 months. What I would say is, the longer you can stick at it, the more likely it will become a habit.

My advice is to start with aiming for 21 days, it really does get easier. If you miss a day, just start again, no judgement. The reward is the reason you will stick at it.

We looked at rewards earlier. Find a reward that works for you and this habit loop will become long term.

So, let's take Cleaning your teeth as an example of a habit.

Cue/Trigger – alarm goes off you get up and head to the bathroom to use the toilet, have a shower and clean your teeth.

Routine – you literally do this every day as part of your morning routine.

Reward – your mouth feels fresh, clean and maybe minty.

Slot your exercise plans into this formula to make it a habit

What exercise could you do to make it a habit? Write your notes here.....

STEP 3 EATING SENSIBLY

Eat better, Feel better

I love food. I love all things sugary in particular sweeties and chocolate. I hate cooking. So, the trick to eating better is to find simple sensible options that work for you.

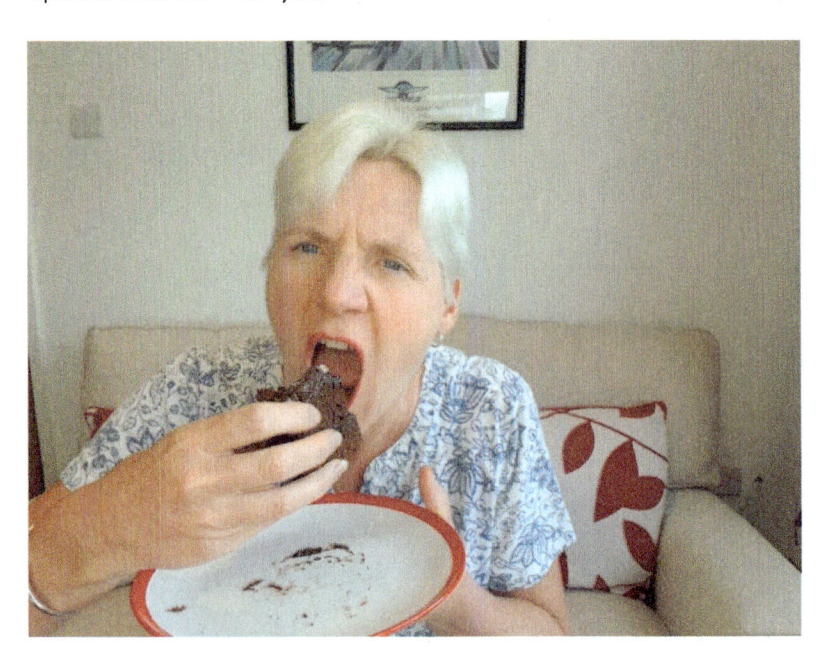

Because I hate cooking, I have had to find meals that I can make that don't have too many ingredients and don't take too long to cook. I have to say, I have made quite a success of this.

I call myself the wok cook; most things get cooked in the wok. If I can get away with just the wok, even better. Although I have now also got a few oven recipes, which are even better as there is practically no washing up after an oven made meal.

I have bought various recipe books over the years but only cooked a handful of the meals. As soon as there is a long list of ingredients, I am put off.

Then they talk about the store cupboard ingredients that you are supposed to have in your cupboards, but I haven't, and I am not buying them for what will inevitably be the only time I make that meal.

A whole selection of my recipe books is a version of lean cooking, but those recipes always look like only half a meal. Whatever your view on carbs, to me a meal is not really a meal without them.

These books talk about pulses, and grains, and non-starchy vegetables. They talk about micro-nutrients and goodness knows what else.

What does that all mean? I don't know and I don't care. I simply want to eat a sensible meal that doesn't take long to make, low effort with good taste.

I do love food,
but I hate thinking about food.
I hate deciding what to cook.

I particularly hate thinking about how many calories it has got and whether it is something I should be eating or not.

I don't count calories anymore; I just make sensible decisions.

I decide what to cook once a week, and then cook those things during the week.

I no longer feel that I am dieting all of the time, I enjoy my food and have a healthy relationship with it, and I still eat cake and ice-cream.

Let me expand on what has worked for me, you can adapt it to suit your life.

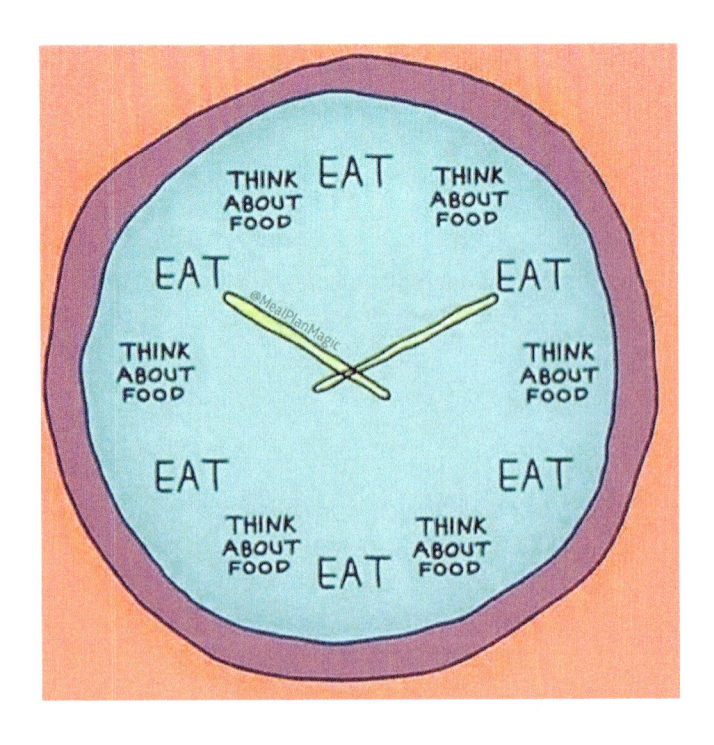

SUGAR RUSH

Stop Snacking. This is the thing that had the single biggest impact on my weight but also changed how I define who I am.

I have always believed that I am a sugar addict. Ever since I was a young girl, I have craved sweets. Where my sister would buy a magazine with her pocket money, I would buy sweets. Where you may drink a glass of wine while you are cooking, I would eat sweets. I jest not.

As I mentioned, I am the person that buys 3 bars of chocolate for £1 at the petrol station, to eat over three days, but then eats them all within a few minutes.

I don't drink tea or coffee and for many years only drunk fruit squash, the sugar version. If I drink alcohol, it will be a sweet wine or a fruity cider. Over a period of many years, I have gradually removed some of these from my diet.

I started drinking water with lemon or cucumber in it and eventually stopped drinking squash completely. I don't even have the salad in it now, just plain water is fine. More than fine, I like water.

In my youth I was a big drinker but as I got older, I just stopped liking it so much. I hardly drink alcohol at all now, which is one thing I don't have to worry about, but maybe you do. I'll come back to drinking in a bit.

Tips to help stop snacking:

Don't buy it!

If only it was that easy, hey?

But seriously, when you shop just don't buy the snacks that pile on the pounds. Avoid the confectionary aisle, or cheese chiller, whatever your weakness is, avoid buying it wherever possible.

If it is not in the house, it takes a lot more effort to go and get it when you start craving it. If other people in the house eat naughty things, get them to hide them away so you can't find them.

OK, so maybe don't hide cheese in the wardrobe, but you get my point. I hide my husband's chocolate biscuits in the salad drawer in the fridge, and as it's not a drawer I go in much (!) I forget about them.

You have to be strong when you are shopping, you know your weakness, don't cave in.

Choose healthy snacks

Swap your fattening snacks for healthier options. Buy nuts, raisons, cherry tomatoes, chopped carrots, rice cakes.

Eat the healthy snacks in moderation, too many nuts are still too fattening, but it stops the sugar craving and only a few will fill you up.

Distract yourself

Snacking is often caused by boredom. The "what can I eat now?" syndrome usually happens when you are doing something you don't want to be doing or you have nothing to do and are bored.

Find something else to distract you, call a friend, make a coffee, watch a funny video, go for a walk around the garden or the block, if you don't have a garden.

You will usually find that once you mind is taken off the snack, you forget about it, for a while anyway.

It is rarely hunger than drives you to want a snack. If I offered you a banana instead of the cake, you'd probably politely decline. It's not hunger, its craving, boredom, habit.

What triggers you to look for a snack? Write your notes here...

What healthy swap could you make? Write your notes here...

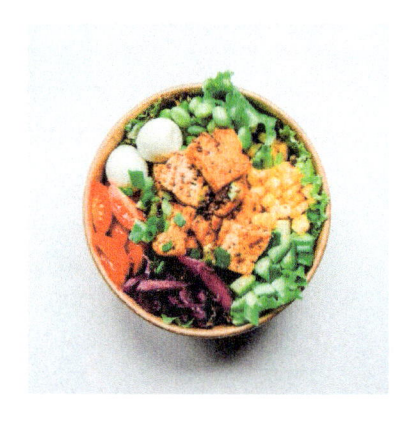

MAKE A MEAL OF IT

Portion size

If you find your plate piled high with food at each meal, then look at reducing your portion size. One trick is to use a smaller plate, so psychologically your brain still sees a full plate. It is amazing at how effective this is.

Dish up a few less carbs, so less potato, chips, rice, bread. Increase the number of vegetables or salad and the protein; the meat, fish, tofu.

We used to have a cooked breakfast every Sunday, it consisted of 2 fried eggs, 2 rashers of bacon, 2 sausages and two slices of toast. When I started wanting to lose weight, I pretty much cut it in half, except the bacon, one bit of bacon is simply not enough. It was still plenty of food and kept us going all day, we didn't miss the additional food. I also swapped fried eggs for poached; a sensible choice.

Three meals a day

It is vital that you do eat regularly. Skipping meals only leads to more snacking and unhealthy choices.

Have a **breakfast** to avoid that mid-morning biscuit craving. Fit it in when it suits you, but do have something, even if it's a banana on the run. I found that taking 5 minutes once I'd got to my desk worked for me.

I was leaving home at 6 am to go to the leisure centre, then heading straight into the office, so I didn't have time for breakfast anywhere else. This meant that I ate it at about 9 am and kept me going until lunch time.

As you will read in a later section, I am not big at food prep but I did start getting into the habit of preparing my breakfast the night before, so I could just grab it in the morning and take it with me, avoiding buying breakfast somewhere or going without.

Lunches have always been the hardest for me, I didn't want a sandwich as I am not a big fan of bread, I find it bloats me.

I don't really rate salad much; I find it dull and boring plus its very seasonal. Who wants a salad in the winter?

I started making what I called a "lunch pot" which was really a bunch of stuff piled in a Tupperware. It was easy because I used whatever was in the fridge, so maybe some ham, a slice of cheese, some cherry tomatoes, a carrot. Or a tin of tuna mixed with a tin of sweetcorn. Prawns with feta, cucumber chunks.

It sort of sounds like a salad, doesn't it, but it didn't feel like salad. I could pick at it when I fancied it.

Just find something that works for you. Maybe you like a sandwich, in which case make a sandwich with wholemeal bread, minimal spread, or use salad cream instead sparingly, add some kind of protein.

You know not to spread the butter thickly or add full fat dressing. You could consider rice cakes or crisp breads with a topping. If you enjoy salad, then great, make a salad but avoid too much creamy coleslaw or salad dressing. Have some but just a small amount.

The biggest action here, is to make your own lunch, don't go and buy it from a shop, because they are full of fattening ingredients. Then don't add the extras, no crisps, chocolate bars etc. Add fruit if you need something else.

Dinner is a meal to be enjoyed in a civilised environment. This is a meal that should be eaten sat at a table, not on your lap. Eating at a table is much better for your digestion which ultimately helps with weight loss.

If you have a family, this is a great time to get everyone together, eat a nice meal and have good conversation. Put your phones away and chat with each other

However, if you have a busy life then this is where dinner becomes a drag.

Deciding what to eat, finding something quick and easy to fit into your busy schedule does not always feel possible. Then it has to be healthy as well, it is just too much trouble.

This is where I decided that I would find myself 9 or 10 meals that I would be able to prep and cook in 30 minutes or less. They would be sensible meals. Not diet meals, healthy meals, lean meals etc, just sensible choices and quick and easy to make.

Let me give you a couple of examples:

I cook a chilli. You could use lamb mince, but beef mince is lower in fat.
I add mushrooms, onions and a pepper. I use a premade packet flavouring. I use these because they are convenient and are mainly natural ingredients. I won't use a sauce from a jar because they are full of sugar and are much more fattening.

I pop it all in the wok and serve with a microwave basmati rice. I can prep and dish up within twenty minutes.

I love a bit of fish, and often eat salmon with roasted veg.

I buy two salmon fillets, I chop a medium potato up into small chunks, along with a red onion, carrot, courgette and a pepper. I put it all on a baking tray with a coating of spray oil and cook for 25 minutes.

One tray of tasty food, and if you really want, you can buy a packet of already chopped veg.

With this meal you could replace the salmon with another type of fish, or a chicken breast or a pork loin.

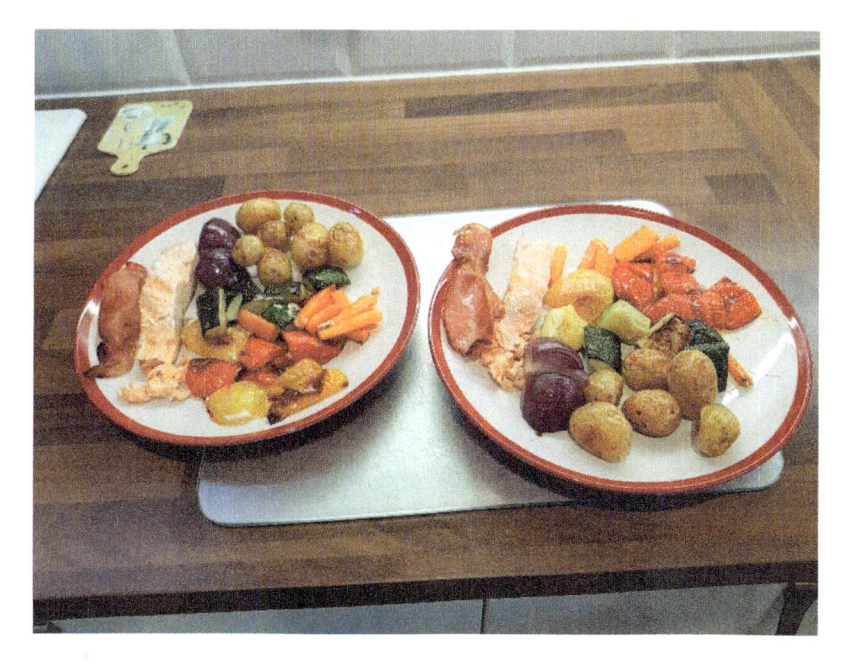

These are just two examples of my easy, sensible choice meals.

Cooking with real ingredients isn't hard if you just learn what works for you and don't overcomplicate it. And that's being said by someone who hates cooking and is not very good at it. As with everything, it gets easier the more you practice. Who knows, maybe you will learn to love cooking.

MIND YOUR FOOD

Mindful eating

Often, we rush eating our meals, we shovel it in without any though at all. This is especially the case with snacks.

Do you ever have those times when you have just eaten a chocolate bar and you actually don't remember eating it?

Or do you eat it in secret, so no-one else knows. Surely if no-one sees you then the calories don't count, right?

The problem is, when you hide it from others, you also hide it from yourself. If you don't remember it, then you just crave more, and so you eat more, and it becomes a never-ending loop of doom.

A bit dramatic, but you understand what I am saying.

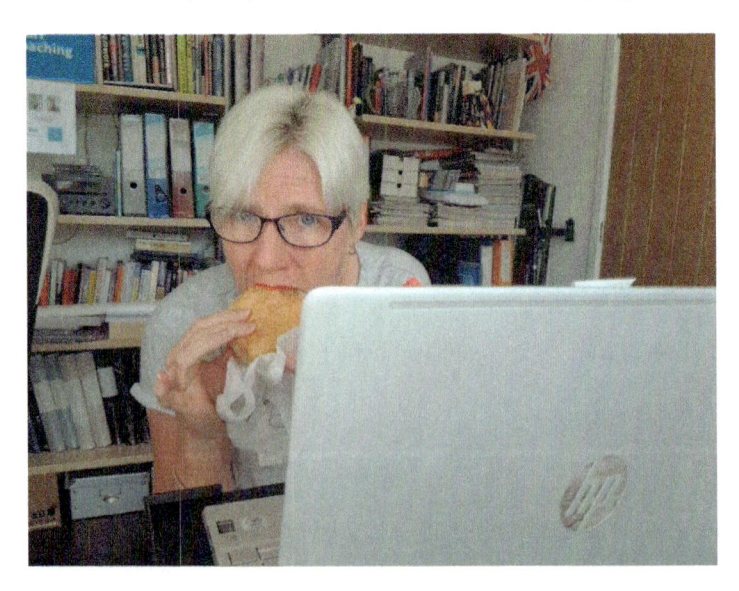

Do you watch the tv when you are eating? I do.

We shouldn't though, because while you are concentrating on what's happening in Albert Square (or your preferred drama) you are not focussing on your food.

Your mind is not even noticing you are eating and so it doesn't tell your brain, or your body and you end up not feeling satisfied.

The trick to feeling full and satisfied is to properly sit and enjoy your meal:

*Sit at a table, sit upright so that your digestive system doesn't have to work so hard.

* Turn off all distractions. Yes, that includes your smart phone. Eat your meal with purpose, chew properly and notice every mouthful.

*Savor the smell, the taste, the consistency. This not only helps your brain realise you are eating, but it actually makes the meal an event to be enjoyed.

I am not suggesting that you never turn on the tv in your kitchen again, or that you adopt a meditative state when you eat. I am just recommending that you find a way to notice what you are eating and enjoy it.

This will make a difference to how much you eat. The more you notice it, the less it will take to fill you up.

Baking

So, I know a lot of you may love doing a bit of baking, and during lockdown people baked a lot.

I am fortunate that I don't like baking but if you are a baker, then this is something you need to address. Either you stop baking, or you keep baking, but you stop eating it.

You could bake and make sure you have people to give it away to.

You could bake smaller cakes, or you could find some lower fat recipes to try.

Cakes, biscuits, pastries etc are extremely good at expanding your waistline and so I would highly recommend that you stop eating them whilst you kickstart your weight loss.

Once you have hit your target you can re-introduce these things in moderation.

Alcohol

Alcohol is a nice accompaniment to a good meal.

Oh, that's not why you drink it?? Well, let's start there. A simple way to reduce your alcohol intake is to replace the wine you drink with your meal, with a glass of water.

Pop the water in a wine glass, it will trick your brain into thinking you are drinking something tasty. You could fill a jug with water and put it on the table, like you get in nice restaurants.

It is all about making things more pleasurable, so you stick with it. If you drink alcohol because you like the taste, then you need to find a way to reduce the amount you drink each week.

Use smaller glasses, limit it to just the weekends, or only when you are out rather than at home.

Any reduction at all will help your weight loss. Look at what type of alcohol you drink, vodka and tonic is less calorific than a pint of lager.

If you drink to **alleviate stress**, then I would really recommend that you find an alternative way.

Yes, alcohol is contributing towards your weight and so reducing it will help with that, but also drinking is never an answer to a stressful situation.

Even though you might think a drink can help you relax, over time, regular drinking will, in fact, interfere with what your brain needs for good mental health, it will impact on your sleep and make stress harder to deal with.

Alcohol disrupts the balance of chemicals in your brain which affects your thoughts, feelings and actions. It is vital that you find other ways to deal with stress, and it's not to reach for food either!

Try things like meditation, exercise, puzzles, singing to your favourite uplifting tune, a hot soak in a bubble bath. I tend to pop on an eighty's song and dance around the kitchen when I feel stressed.

Another thing is to laugh, find a comedy programme to watch and have a good belly laugh.

Water

Drink more water.

Often when we think we are hungry, we are actually dehydrated. Aim to drink 2 litres of water each day. Get a water bottle so you can have it to hand wherever you are, just get into the habit of filling it and drinking from it.

I find when I get towards the end of my walk each morning that I am feeling hungry, but when I get home and glug a glass of water, the feeling goes away.

Drinking water is a healthy thing to do anyway but it definitely helps in the weight loss arena.

Drink before you eat your meal, it will fill you up.

Drink before you go shopping so you don't feel hungry.

Drink when you feel like a snack.

All of these simple actions will help you lose weight. Even if you only do some of them, any reduction in food will help you shed the pounds. It is all about having that positive thinking and making sensible choices.

Sensible choice examples:

Bad choice	Better choice
Sugary cereal	Porridge oats
Battered fish	Breaded fish
Chips	New potatoes
White bread	Wholemeal bread
Sticky pudding	Fruit and yogurt
Chocolate bar	Handful of raisins
Magnum ice lolly	Solero ice lolly
Glass of wine	Small glass of champagne

What could you change to make more sensible food choices? Write your notes here...

STEP 4 – PLANNING

Prepare for success

Some kind of planning and preparation will definitely help you achieve your goals and makes it easier to stick to your positive **thin**king approach.

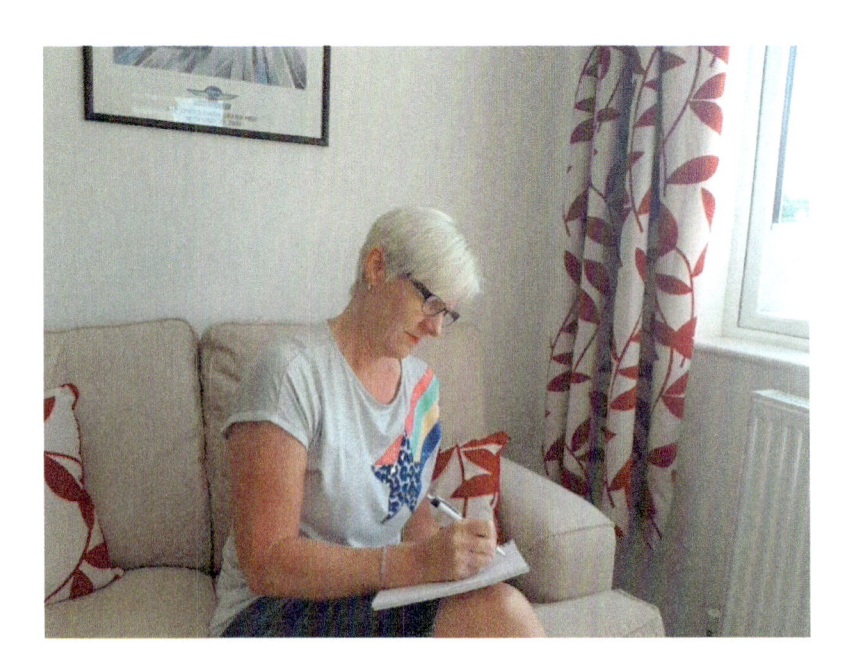

I like a bit of a plan, a loose plan but not too much detail.

I get bogged down in detail and I am not big on preparation in life.

Obviously, there are exceptions, if I am doing a presentation or going for an interview etc then preparation is key, but even then, I only go so far, I am definitely not a perfectionist. There is always an element of "winging it' in my life.

If I am doing a dinner party…. hang on, that sounds grand, I don't have dinner parties, but occasionally my parents come round for dinner…..then there will be some planning and preparation involved, particularly as I am not a confident cook.

The less confident you are at something, the more I would recommend planning for it. It removes some of the stress of being outside your comfort zone if you have done your prep.

Let me give you an example of something just this week.

I had been thinking that I need to increase my strength and a class popped up on Facebook for strength training, just down the road at the local community centre.

I booked to go, then that afternoon I started to feel nervous about going. I was going on my own, I wouldn't know anyone there, I didn't know what it would be like, would I be able to do it?

But I had my kit all ready, I knew exactly where it was being held, how long it would take me to get there, where to park and what room the session was in. I decided, I had nothing to lose, I only had to go once and if I didn't like it, I wouldn't go again.

I did go but if I hadn't prepared earlier in the day, I may well have chickened out.

Planning for eating

Let's look at how to plan and prepare for success with sensible eating.

Menu

My top tip here is to plan a menu for the week.

This way you know what you will be eating each day, no reason for indecisiveness to lead to bad choices.

Plan your menu around your schedule. So, if you know you will be working late one evening, that day you have a quick to make meal. If you know you are eating out one lunchtime, then you plan for a lighter meal that evening.

You don't need to decide exactly which day you eat the meals, but at least choose 7 main meals, 7 lunches and 7 breakfasts. Make sure they are meals that fit into your lifestyle, otherwise the food will get left to go stale or mouldy while you get a takeaway.

Plan in your snacks. If you feel you will still need some kind of snack, then buy something as a healthy alternative to the sugary kind.

Going shopping once a week means that you can buy fresh food to last the week and stops the need to waste time shopping more than once a week. I can do my weekly shop in 45 minutes now.

Shopping list

Write your shopping list from this menu plan, note down the date, so that when you are shopping you can buy items that are within their used by date.

Only buy these ingredients when you are in the shop, don't get tempted by other sparkly objects.

Don't go shopping when you are hungry, in fact, shopping when you have eaten and are full up is best, it stops the cravings show up. At least have a glass of water to fill your belly before shopping.

Choose fresh produce wherever possible, and preferably loose, not packaged if possible. Let's try and save the planet a little while we are at it.

Food prep

Now, some people swear by a full food prep session, where they batch cook meals for the week on a Sunday. If this works for you, the be my guest, go for it.

Personally, I do not want to spend a few hours on my Sunday playing with my food. I would much rather just cook each day; my meals are not time consuming so spreading my time over the week works much better for me.

However, I have found a couple of preparation tricks that do work for me. They were particularly useful when I was leaving the house every day to work in an office.

I would always prepare breakfast the night before. I left home early to go to the gym, so I didn't eat at home before I went, and I needed to have something I could eat at my desk.

I had a few go-to breakfasts, but my favourite was fruit and yogurt. Banana sliced at the bottom of a Tupperware bowl, covered with natural fat free yogurt and topped with berries. And a lunch which I would also make the night before, salad, sandwich, snack pot. Then they would both go in a cool bag and in the fridge overnight for me to literally grab and take with me in the morning.

The other preparation worth considering is the snacks. If you want some fruit to munch on during the day, then peel and chop before-hand, stick in a Tupperware or a sealable food bag to enjoy when you fancy it. A chopped-up apple is, somehow, much tastier than a whole one.

The biggest impact with sensible eating is simply to **plan** *what you will be eating each day and having the right ingredients to hand. This will ensure it is easy to make the right choices and will stop you going astray.*

What food planning could you do? Write your notes here....

PLANNING FOR EXERCISE

When and where

Once you have decided which exercise works for you, then plan it in. Whether that's doing it as soon as you get up, or after work, plan it in and stick to it.

* If you are going to a class or a group session, then make sure you know where and when it is, how to get there, where to park etc. If you can go with a buddy who is equally as committed to making a change then that can really spur you to go each week.

* If you are exercising at home, have the dvd, download, online class ready for you to get going when you are ready. Set up the appropriate space, whether that's your bedroom, living room or garden, you don't want to be having to clear things away to get started, this will just stop you doing it.

* If you are going out to exercise under your own steam, so walking, running or cycling then plan your route, at least to start with. Once you have been out a few times you will know where you are going but those first occasions can be daunting if you haven't been out on your own before.

* One option would be to rope in a friend, partner, child to go and scope out the best place to go before hand. Have a look for your local park, woods, sea front or just some quiet roads. Starting your exercise from home is always best but if you have to drive somewhere, then even more reason to investigate the best place and do a trial run. I find if I have to get in the car, it is just another barrier to stop me doing it.

* If you are using your treadmill, static bike or any other home gym equipment, then make sure you have removed all the clothes hanging on it, so it's free to use!

Kit

Always have your kit ready. Know what you need.

If it's a class, do you need a floor mat or to have your hair tied back?

For most exercise you only need a pair of trainers, some comfy jogging bottoms or shorts and a t' shirt, and maybe a sports bra.

You don't need nice new kit, use what you have hanging around in your wardrobe. I have jogging bottoms that I have had longer than I have known my husband and that's over 25 years. My trainers are falling apart but they still do the job, and my sports bra only has two hooks out of three still hanging on in there.

Once you have pulled your kit out, have it ready to pull on at the time you have decided you are exercising. My kit is piled on a chair beside my bed which I put on as soon as I get up. My trainers are right by the door to slip my feet into on my way out. They are pretty much held together by mud, so they don't come any further into the house.

Other people

It's a good idea to tell anyone else in your household when you are going to be busy with your exercise. It should be made clear to them that this is your time, its important to you and you would really appreciate their support in enabling this to happen.

In fact, this is a good thing to do for both your exercise and eating plans. One of the biggest things that sabotages us is other people in our lives, who either don't support your plans or who just don't get it.

If you are lucky enough to have a supportive family, partner and friends then explain to them what you are doing, why you are doing. Share with them the impact it will have on your life to make this change and ask them to help make it easy for you.

If the people in your inner circle are not so supportive, whether they are critical or just don't know how to be supportive, then my advice would be to carry on quietly without disturbing them too much.

Remind yourself that this is all about **YOU**, how you want to improve yourself and feel better. Just keep your head down and get on with making sensible choices.

I haven't always told my husband when am changing what I do, I just get on with it, and when he asks why I haven't eaten a biscuit, I just say that I didn't fancy one, or that I was full up from dinner.

What planning could you do? Write your notes here...

CELEBRATION

Progress not perfection

The final part of this process is to remember to celebrate your success. Notice every tiny little win you have and celebrate it. Give yourself a gold star or a pat on the back.

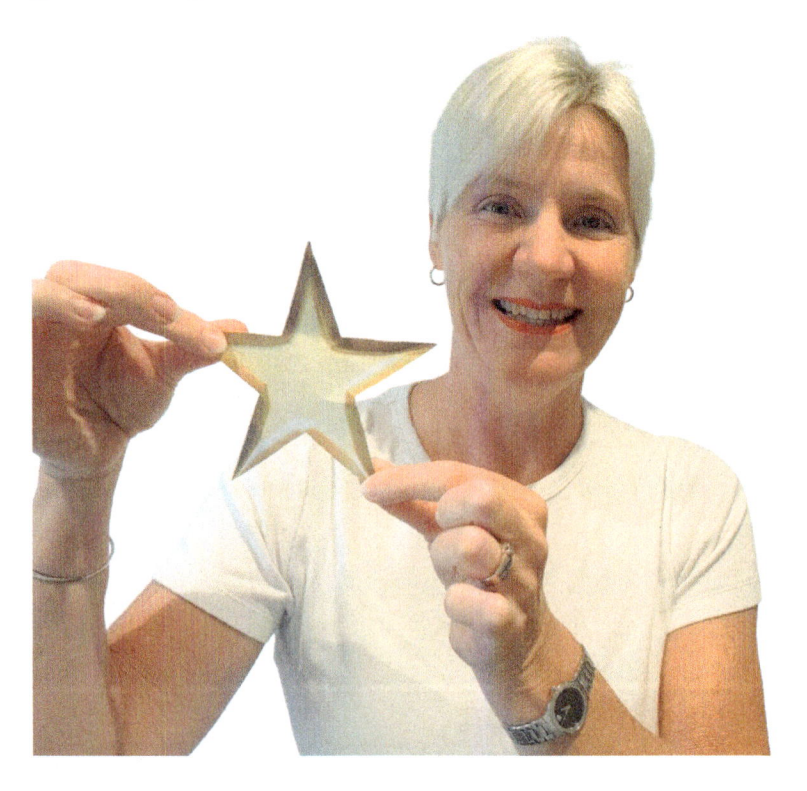

Don't celebrate with champagne and chocolate cake.

Seriously though, you will have good days and bad days.

You will have times where it feels easy and the weight falls off, and you will have periods where it feels impossible, and the stubborn pounds simply don't shift.

This is normal, but don't give up. If you lapse one day, don't beat yourself up, just start again the next day. One bad day will only impact on you if it becomes two, three, ten bad days.

At times like this revisit your visualisations – remember how bad you feel being fat and how good you will feel being the new you.

Reflect and review

Every day take some time to pause and reflect on what went well, recognise the good choices that you made and congratulate yourself for those moments.

Only look at the good things, train your brain to realise that you are doing well and it is possible to achieve your goals. It is important to reward the effort you are making, even if you don't hit the goal, as long as you have made progress, that's great.

Sometimes progress, will be not having put on any weight, this is still good. Ask yourself:

Did you do the best you could today?

What will you do differently tomorrow?

Weigh in

I would recommend that you weigh yourself once a week at the same time wearing the same clothes, or no clothes. A week is enough time to have made a difference and gives you regular feedback on where you are in your weight loss journey.

Do not weigh yourself every day, this is pointless and often depressing. If you find you have put on a lb or 2, just adapt your menu for the following week and keep that positive thinking and visualise the new you.

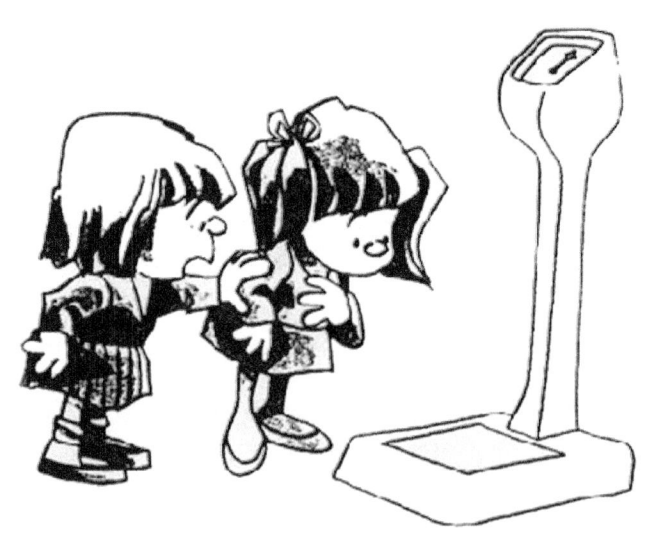

"Don't step on it...it will make you cry."

Not losing weight?

If you find its not working and you are not losing any weight, then there are two things to consider:

1) Are you being honest with yourself?

   Are you still eating snacks but not admitting it?

   Have you missed a few days exercise because you are too busy?

You must be honest, the only person you are misleading is **YOU**, and the only person it is impacting is **YOU**.

Try writing a food diary and list absolutely everything you are eating, no matter how small. This will soon identify where you could make changes.

You could also have an exercise schedule that you tick off to show you how often you have missed a day.

2) Are there things that are not suiting you?

   Do some foods bloat you?

   Do you hate the exercise you are doing?

In these cases, try something else.

It will often be a case of trial and error before you find what works for you.

I have been trying things for over ten years to get to my sweet spot. **Don't give up**, just find different choices that suit you and your lifestyle.

Motivation

Make a chart with your goals on it that you can add stars to.

When you have had a good day, pop a gold star on your chart, see how many good days you have.

Another option is to have a funky visual goal. So, maybe draw a large picture of a person, a dress, a cake and add small sections that equal a pound (lb).

As you lose weight, you can colour the chart in. Having a visual image to see how well you are doing can be very motivating.

I always look forward to colouring in another section or ticking off a day where I didn't eat any sugar.

Whichever way you do it, find a way to notice all the good steps you make, congratulate yourself and celebrate every small success you achieve. Every time you celebrate, you are telling your brain how capable you are.

You are giving it positive messages which leads to affirmation that you are awesome.

You are looking for ***progress not perfection***.

Progress leads to traction and motivation and ultimately to more progress. Once you are on this roll, you will start to gather momentum and things will start to become a habit, a lifestyle and just who you are.

Say after me: "**I am committed to becoming slim, healthy and happy, because I deserve it**"

FEELING FABULOUS

Slim, Fit and Happy

I want to end this book by trying to explain to you how amazing you will feel when you crack this. I now love who I see in the mirror.

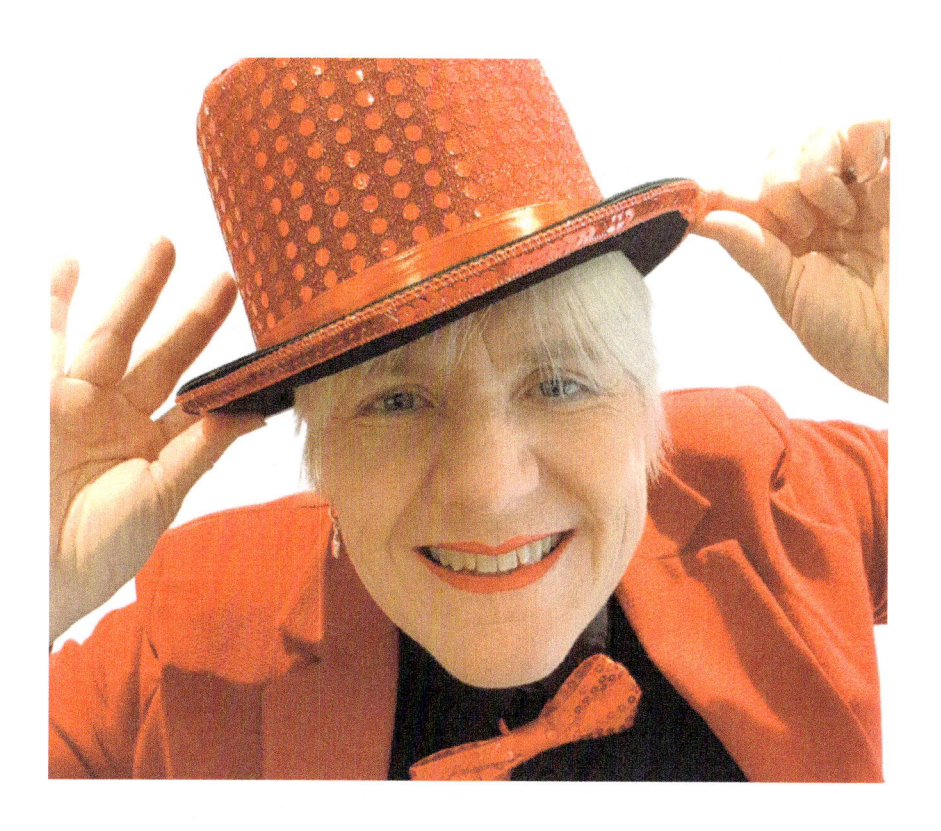

I like the look of my body. In fact, when I get up every morning, I am looking forward to seeing myself in the mirror. I blow myself a kiss and smile at how great I look.

I am not perfect, by any means. I still have wobbly thighs and my tummy is not completely flat but that's OK. I am happy with how I am, and I love what I see so much that I find it easy to make the right choice.

You need to decide what you will be happy with and when you arrive there, enjoy it. Notice it, love it, feel it. It will keep you motivated to maintain the lifestyle you have made for yourself.

I don't spend any energy thinking about food. I plan my food once a week, then just cook and eat according to my plan.

I know what my sensible choices are, and I now know how to enjoy food without feeling guilty or disappointed in myself. It is very liberating, not having to focus on food so much.

I am not always sensible; I do have lapses, but I know that I can get back on track easily using these steps.

I feel fabulous. I am no longer stodgy and lacking in energy. I don't slump and shuffle. I have so much energy now, I am ready for the day when I get up.

I love my 5 mile walk every morning and my tasty, healthy breakfast. I am performing better in my life and in my business. I can take on new challenges and not feel overwhelmed by them.

My focus and energy have improved by removing sugar and processed food from my diet

My fitness has improved due to the exercise and at 52 I feel the slimmest, fittest and happiest that I have ever felt. *I am more confident; I feel very capable and I am living a happy fulfilling life.*

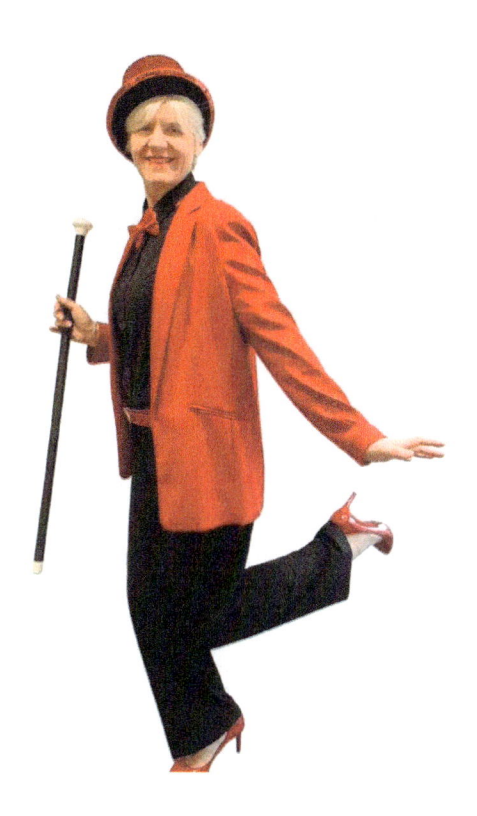

I want this for you too, so one quick summary and then you just need to take that first step.

1. **DECIDE** – Change your mindset by understanding what you want and why you want it. Get yourself in that Positive **thin**king mode and get committed to make a lifestyle change

2. **EXERCISE** – Find something that you enjoy and want to do, but at a minimum, just MOVE MORE

3. **EAT SENSIBLY** – Make sensible choices, drink less and stop snacking.

4. **PLAN** – Plan what you are going to eat, so you only eat what you buy. Plan your exercise so that you make it a habit.

5. **CELEBRATE** – Notice every small win, celebrate your progress and keep the momentum going.

⭐ positive **thin**king is all it takes

Now you have all that you need to make the change to your life. BUT will you?

Now that you have you read this book all the way through, will you take action, or will you pop it on the shelf to gather dust?

Remember, the only person standing in your way is **YOU**.

- ❖ Do you need some help?

- ❖ Do you need someone to motivate you, to get you started and help you get into that positive thinking mode?

- ❖ Maybe you need someone to help you track your progress and give you little pep talks, someone to hold you to account.

- ❖ Perhaps you need a cheerleader, someone who will celebrate with you when you make progress.

Whatever you need to become the person you deserve to be, go and find it.

I would love to help you on your journey, and if you think I am the person to help you then give me a shout………

Reach out to the Starr.

To work with Sheila:

* email her at sheila@sheilastarrcoaching.co.uk

Connect with Sheila on LinkedIn:
www.linkedin.com/in/sheila-starr

Like and follow her on Facebook:
@sheilastarr69

Sheila also has a Facebook group to help inspire women to thrive:

www.facebook.com/groups/sheilastarrinspiringwomentothrive

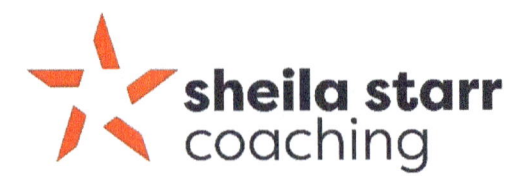

sheila starr coaching

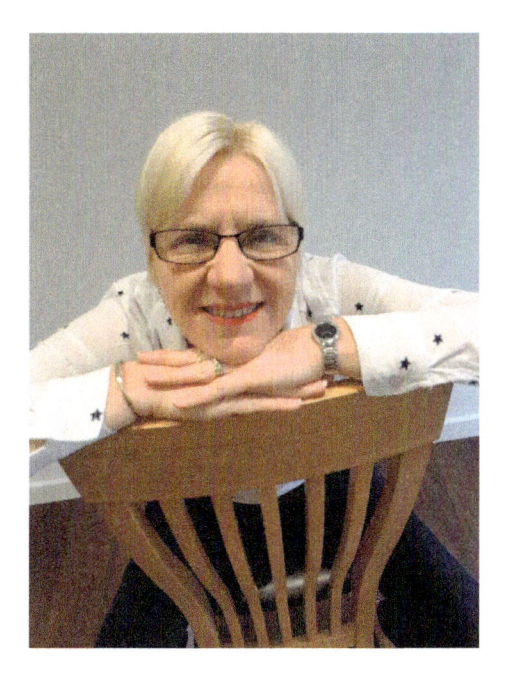

Sheila lives in Eastleigh on the South Coast of England with her husband. She has worked in corporate life for over 30 years setting up and running customer service and transformation teams. She has spent a lot of time coaching and mentoring and now runs her own coaching business. Sheila is passionate about helping people live happy, fulfilling lives, and to love who they are.

Printed in Great Britain
by Amazon